Fructose -
The Evil Twin

Sweet And Deadly

Rudy Kachmann M.D.

Contents

Preface

YOU MAY HAVE THOUGHT THAT the original evil twins were insulin resistance and inflammation, the cause of most of our chronic disease and type 2 diabetes, vascular disease, heart disease, strokes, autoimmune disease and cancer.

However, those two are the children of the fraternal twins, glucose and fructose.

Sucrose, or table sugar, is 50% glucose and 50% fructose. Their chemical configuration is identical: $C_6H_{12}O_6$. They are twins. However, they are metabolized in the body totally differently. Even though they are isomer (mirror images) of each other, our bodies recognize them differently. One of them is chemically a hexagon and the other a pentagon.

After digestion, glucose heads for the bloodstream and we use it for energy, in the muscles, brain, liver and what's left over is converted to glycogen and sometimes fat. Fructose goes straight to the liver and raises havoc, leading to insulin resistance, leptin resistance, inflammation, fatty liver, and very low density lipoprotein (VLDL), which is the cause of atherosclerosis, dementia, some forms of cancer and many other illnesses.

This book will explain how to avoid these evil twins and prevent most chronic diseases, allowing you to lead a healthy life, increase your energy levels, look great and live to be a 100 or more.

FRUCTOSE - THE EVIL TWIN

Fructose is the "evil dragon" and I will teach you how to identify, avoid and, if necessary, fight and destroy him.

Let's get going on our venture.

Taking Back Our Health

WE'RE HAVING A NATIONAL AND international epidemic of obesity, type 2 diabetes, heart disease, vascular disease, strokes and cancer. The China Study by Dr. Colin Campbell certainly pointed us in that direction. The United States has the second-highest rate of obesity in the world, only second to Mexico. It's about fat salt and sugar with sugar being the main culprit.

Each year, Americans suffer 1.5 million heart attacks, including 850,000 deaths from heart attacks, 35 million people have type 2 diabetes, and 125 million people have metabolic syndrome, in addition to some of the highest rates of cancer in the world and essentially leading the world in chronic disease. Seventy-five percent of us are overweight, 35 to 40% are obese, one third of our children are overweight -- from those figures, you can predict the future.

This is a no judgment zone; I'm just trying to help solve the problem that is killing us.

History

WE'VE BEEN EXPOSED TO AN avalanche of diets: the Atkins Diet, low carb and high protein, Paleo, Pritikin, vegetarian, Dr. Dean Ornish, essentially vegetarian, Dr. Caldwell Esseltyne, Dr. Joel Fuhrman, 80% high density nutrient, 20% low-fat meat products, Dr. Richard Young, sugar-fix, Dr. Rosedale diet, leptin control, etc. I've read about them all. Frankly, there's something good in all of them, although I don't agree with everything. There clearly is no "best" diet.

Personally, I think a combination of Dr. Robert Lustig, Dr. Joel Fuhrman, Dr. Caldwell Esseltyne, Dr. Dean Ornish, Dr. Kachmann, my book "Secret of the Non-Diet", and especially Dr. Richard Johnson's book, "The Sugar Fix" and the Dr. Ron Rosedale's diet hit the mark. I quote from them liberally.

Dr. Robert Lustig in his famous book, New York Times bestseller, "Fat Chance," and Dr. Richard Johnson emphasize the evil twin fructose as the main culprit for our declining health. I agree.

What I witnessed in working at hospitals for 44 years was the horrible complications of vascular disease, heart attacks, strokes, cancer as a result of improper eating and obesity, all of which are incredibly sad. There is great hope because these chronic illnesses are largely preventable and many can be stopped, prevented and reversed. I have seen it. I have taught it!

We need to participate in our healthcare, what we have now is "sick care." We need to speak to our patients, read, research and ask for the help of our families and providers. The wellness wheel begins with participating in your healthcare.

We need to understand the physiology of fructose, what foods contain it and what foods to eat, plus other good health habits like exercise and stress reduction to enjoy a healthy happy life.

In this book you will learn about good carbohydrates, proteins and fats. Yes, fat is not quite the enemy you thought it was, as part of the problem, sugar, is the real toxin.

The White Menace

EVERY SUCCESSFUL DIET RESTRICTS SUGAR, but, as Dr. Lustig says, that is the Lex Luther of the story. Sugar is both a carbohydrate, which a lot of it comes from, as well as a fat, where it can end up if it is not used. These twins, **glucose and fructose,** are the evil ones. Many people are addicted to sugar, and many say that it is as addictive as cocaine.

As already mentioned their chemical formula is the same, but they are metabolized differently.

They affect our mental state by influencing our appetite center, and affect our serotonin and dopamine circuitry. They act like cocaine or heroin and cause the "bliss point" of desire -- the quick fix, the sugar fix. No matter how hard you try, if you don't fix the sugar problem, you won't lose weight. Sugar makes you fat and sick if you consume enough of it

The industrial complex, Cargill, Kellogg, Hershey etc., figured out this bliss point. The Monell Company in Philadelphia, financed by industry and the government studies, knows exactly the amount of sugar and fat it takes to light up our brain with pleasure. They know what foods are most palatable to us. Sales are dependent on it. That's where fast food comes from. They know your bliss point for sugar and adults is 26% and 38% for teenagers. That knowledge is killing us. Children's brains are more easily addicted to sugar, because they're not fully developed.

You've heard of empty calories, calories without nutrients, vitamins, minerals and phytochemicals, and certainly sugar has none of these. Many of us are addicted to sugar but it's the fructose that has a special payload because of its effect on the liver.

Fructose actually is the main sugar in fruit, which we all know, that is good for us! Wrong! In reasonable quantities, consumed in its original form, with fiber and no more than 35 grams daily, it's quite healthy. Fruit juice has more fructose than high fructose corn syrup. But fructose in fruit is not that much metabolically different than the fructose and sucrose in corn syrup, to my dismay. To my surprise, excess fruit consumption can have its problems, too. We prefer fructose because it is sweet, it hits the bliss point.

Industry knows how to make it from corn syrup, and recognized that it is sweeter than regular sucrose and cheaper, making a lot of money because of it. Just read the book "Fat, Salt and Sugar" by reporter Michael Moss. High fructose corn syrup was invented by the Japanese in the late 1960s and its consumption has skyrocketed. Today, it is at least 50 to 75% of the cause of our obesity and chronic disease problems. Just look around in a public place, it's plain scary. Many people think this epidemic is genetic when actually it is the reaction of our bodies to the sugar epidemic.

We consume 6.5 ounces of sugar a day, and 130 pounds a year, including about 50 pounds of fructose yearly. We have increased our fructose consumption five-fold in 100 years. The CDC says 50% of us are consuming at least one fructose drink a day, and 10% drink three or more daily.

Sugar has infiltrated thousands of manufactured foods we see in the major markets. Much of our consumption actually comes from manufactured food combinations, and 20% of our calories come from sugar products. We consume 20 teaspoons full of sugar daily. Some of our teenagers are consuming 30 to 40% of their calories from sugar. It's occurring all over the world.

I read in the newspaper the other day that Mexico just surpassed us in obesity, which puts us in the number 2 spot in the western world. They imposed a 10% sales tax on sugary sodas, and an 8% tax on fast food. From what I know about the economic formula called the elasticity of demand that will not change the behavior of the people, although it's a good start. Vietnam, South Korea and Asia are all reporting high rates of type 2 diabetes and obesity. Many have restaurants with the same name and you can see the problem. Fat, salt and sugar. The global consumption of sugar has increased 50%.

The American Heart Association recommends 150 sugar calories a day for men and 100 calories a day for women, but we are blowing past that at around 500-600 calories.

We'd all like to blame high fructose corn syrup as being the main devil, but actually that is only partially true. Fructose is fructose, yes, even from fruit. Fiber keeps us from absorbing some of the sugar, but fructose is still fructose.

High fructose corn syrup consumption is going down because of government laws, but it's a public health problem and we need stronger national laws. At least we have started to control trans-fats and we could do the same for fructose by limiting it. Meanwhile, obesity rate continues to increase. It's the "evil twin" at work.

My friend Dr. Joel Fuhrman was hired to teach proper nutrition in South Korea because of the obesity and type 2 diabetes problem. He told me all about it when I was with in Italy recently.

Dr. Robert Lustig says in his famous book "Fat Chance" that scientific evidence supports the notion that HFCS is actually no different from sucrose, although high fructose corn sugar does generate a higher blood fructose level, which could have metabolic consequences. But the difference is small, 10 to 15%.

Dr. Lustig says that sugar in any form is toxic. I say fructose is just the evil twin of its malignant brother, glucose. All sugar is potentially toxic and I completely agree with Dr. Lustig. Calorie for calorie, orange juice is worse for you than soda. Orange juice has 1.8 grams of fructose; soda has 1.7 g of fructose, according to Dr.Lustig.

Twin Metabolism: Glucose and Fructose

THE EVIL TWIN, FRUCTOSE, IS separated from his brother glucose in the gut and heads for the bloodstream. It doesn't raise the insulin level like glucose and without insulin enters the liver cells and starts its evil path of destruction. Fructose, incidentally, is never found in nature without being chemically attached to something else. It's always attached to his brother glucose.

Fructose causes the browning reaction like you see in frying, or what's known as the formation of AGEs, advanced glycation end products.

When glucose attaches to protein in the blood, it can wreak havoc in the body, contributing to aging and chronic disease. The HBA 1C is an example in which we are determining the blood sugar level over a three-month period. That's why fruit turns brown and becomes a lot sweeter. It's called the Mailard reaction and is seven times faster than the glucose reaction. This drives the aging process in many degenerative diseases, like arthritis, dementia, cancer, heart disease, breast disease and autoimmune disease.

Fructose leads to inflammation and insulin resistance. The liver metabolizes 95% of fructose and the kidney metabolizes 5%. Let's review the steps of fructose metabolism.

The liver needs three times as much energy to metabolize fructose as it does for glucose. Metabolism is defined as the sum of the chemical activity necessary to carry out a reaction. That depletes the level of ATP, adenosine triphosphate, our energy molecule in the mitochondria of our cells. The mitochondria are little energy factories, which every cell has – there are about 10,000 factories per cell, and trillions in the human body. No mitochondria, no energy. The waste product of ATP metabolism is uric acid and purines, which cause hypertension. That's the reason type 2 diabetics all have high blood pressure.

It goes straight to acetyl-coA, exceeding the mitochondria's ability to metabolize it. The acetyl-coA converts the energy of fructose to fat. The fat is deposited mainly in the liver and causes non-alcoholic fatty liver disease, NAFLD. This results in insulin resistance, leptin resistance and inflammation. Leptin is a hormone of fat that regulates fat deposition, appetite and is the king of hormones. If you have leptin resistance, you get fat and it doesn't turn off your appetite like high sugar would without insulin resistance.

Fructose then activates a liver enzyme, which causes inflammation throughout the body, resulting in heart disease, strokes, dementia, cancer and autoimmune disease.

We could not live without glucose. It makes ATP with oxygen, the energy molecule. Twenty percent of our glucose is used for brain fuel, although ketones from fat metabolism can be used by the brain. Glucose without fructose is called starch, a friendly food source.

When we consume sugar, 20% or so goes to the liver and is converted to glycogen, 80% hits the bloodstream and is utilized for energy by the brain, liver metabolism and muscle.

Glucose metabolism is completely dependent on insulin; it can't enter cells without it. Sugar has a great effect on our brain and some people think it's more addictive than narcotics. Any excess glucose in the liver that's not converted to glycogen or used to create energy will be converted to fat. Yes, glucose and fructose can make you fat, fructose is just a lot worse.

Also glucose can bind to protein, releasing a free radical, an electron, which can destroy your body when in excess. That is called oxidation. It is also called a reactive oxygen species-ROS. They can cause a lot of our chronic diseases and need to be removed.

We are FRUCKED

MANY OTHER PRIMATES CAN EXIST on vegetables and fruit alone, have long intestines like us and develop little chronic disease. In nature, fructose intake is limited.

Our ancestors ate only about 20 to 25% fruit in their diet and it was all seasonal. They did not eat additional sugar like so many of us do today.

Sugar is a big player but that 50% is fructose is the lion on the field. Sedentary lifestyles and too much animal protein loaded with saturated fat are also a part of the problem. Gluten sensitivity can contribute to this issue and should be tested in everyone.

Physiology of the Evil Twin and His Brother

JOHN YUDKIN (1910- 1995) TRIED to warn us about sugar. He lost the food fight to Ansell Keys for about 30 years, but his knowledge is now leading the race.

Yudkin, a British physiologist and nutritionist, became internationally famous with this book "Pure, White and Deadly" in 1972. He was one of the first scientists to claim that sugar was a major cause of obesity and heart disease.

I think Dr. Robert H.Lustig, a pediatric endocrinologist from the division of endocrinology at the University of California, San Francisco, has republished Dr. Yudkin's book as I see his name on the cover. I thank him for that.

For a few decades it was thought that fat was the main culprit in poor health, but the tide is turning.

In his introduction Dr.Lustig says, "everything old is new again." I was hoping he was talking about me. I'm having my 39th celebration of my 39th birthday next year.

Ansell Keys, the University of Minnesota epidemiologist, stated that saturated fat was the main cause of vascular disease in 1953. He published the seven countries study.

Dr.Lustig says three scientific findings undid the Yudkin case.

By studying the genetic disease of familial hypercholester-olemia, where people at a very young age had very abnormal blood studies, Dr. Michael Brown and Dr. Joseph Goldstein discovered low-density lipoprotein LDL and the LDL receptor, leading to the hypothesis that LDL was the bad actor. We now know that it is very low-density LDL from fructose that is the devil that is killing us. They did not know that at that time and that is what undid Dr. Yudkin. So the fight began and Yudkin was run over by the "fat theory" people. They were wrong.

Additional large studies begin to demonstrate that triglycerides correlated more with sugar consumption. Also, the discovery that very low-density LDL, VLDL was driven by diet, sugar and especially fructose started to change people's thinking about the "fat theory" and Ansell Keyes.

Low Carbohydrate Diets

LOW CARBOHYDRATE DIETS CAME TO the forefront, including the Atkins and Paleo diets. In addition, Syndrome X, metabolic syndrome, was described by Dr. Raven.

Dr. Lustig ran across the Yudkin work at a meeting in 2008 and has been a champion ever since (although he was ready doing a great deal of research on sugar and felt it was the real culprit). I think Dr. Lustig is a champion of the sugar fructose debate as well as Dr. Richard Johnson as described in his book "Sugar Fix." They have the answer as far as I'm concerned; I'm just trying to bring the point home because I'm a wellness teacher.

You now know that things have advanced since Dr. Yudkin and the causation is well described by Dr. Richard Johnson and Dr. Lustig. Sugar is addictive and affects the psychology of many people, and it is ruining their health. It affects the serotonin dopamine circuitry of addiction. Dr.Lustig says he is a Yudkin disciple. Put me on the list!

Sugar is the answer to food addiction; if avoided, most people can achieve a normal weight and great health.

The Evil Twin Revisited

DR. YUDKIN, DR.LUSTIG AND DR. Richard Johnson have advanced the research, education, publication and treatment of chronic disease that is killing us. Many others have written books along the way, including Dr. Dean Ornish, Dr. Joel Fuhrman, Dr. McDougall, Dr. Caldwell Esseltyne of the Cleveland Clinic, Dr. Neal Bernard, Dr. Hans Diehl, and my own books and have helped advance prevention, reversing the treatment of vascular disease, diabetes, cancer prevention, autoimmune disease and more.

The beauty is that the enemy is in our sites and can be killed with one shot: Avoid the evil twin fructose.

Just sit in a restaurant, at a ballgame or school and look at the size of the people. I've been sitting at Starbucks today for more than two hours while writing this. The restaurant across the way is even worse. This is a no-judgment zone, but were not going to solve this problem if we don't really look at it. The same problem is occurring across the world.

In 1890, 5% of Americans were obese. Now it's greater than 35%, plus the 75 to 80% who are overweight. Certain ethnic and racial groups are even approaching 90%.

It's alarming, sickly and costly. Health education is poor; people are eating government-supported genetically altered food. What they do to animals to put them on your plate is beyond comprehension. Milk and cheese products are full of saturated fats, which adds to the problem. Food stamps have no nutrient requirements and are killing people. The poor have a much worse obesity rate because the government-supported food they're eating is influenced by politics and lobbying rather than a focus on good health. Certainly, obesity is psychologically crippling to many people and especially children. A lot of people think it's genetic in origin when it's truly the reaction of the genes to what people are eating. Sometimes a whole family eats the wrong food because they are not aware of what they're doing to themselves, so providers and educators must get more seriously involved.

The government should not support the prices of fat, salt and sugar. They should support organic farming and gardening. I think it's more of what we eat and the amount we are eating. I don't think calorie counting is necessary: Simply eat the right food and exercise 30 minutes a day. We are consuming the evil twin 30% more than in 1970 and that parallels our increase in obesity rates.

Fructose is the main sugar in fruit and has been for 1 million years. Our ancient ancestors and primate animals lived on that. But they exercised a lot and they needed to store fat to survive, so fructose didn't cause the diseases we are seeing.

Some people call high fructose corn syrup "Frankensyrup." It's cheap and sweet and deadly.

In summary, avoiding fructose is a good start on great health. The next few chapters explain how to do it. In addition I would view some other aspects of gluten, which some people are sensitive to as well as saturated fat.

Food Stamp Diet

THE PEOPLE USING FOOD STAMPS are, on the average, more overweight than the rest of us. The country is running about 70% overweight. Our leadership doesn't even bring it up and allows more people to develop a high rate of chronic disease and early death. I do a lot of charitable work in my community, including being a sponsor of a large choir and I am very familiar with it and trying to help the best I can. I write books, CDs, DVDs, participate on a TV show and give frequent lectures about the problem and I think am making some difference.

A first reaction might be that good food is more expensive and there isn't enough money. Really? The majority of people on food stamps don't look like they're starving; it's just the opposite. I give cooking classes with a pediatrician, Dr. Gary Verulla, once a month and about 90% of his patients are on food stamps. When I visit his waiting room, I would say 90% of the mothers and children are seriously overweight.

We're doing something about it by offering cooking classes and the children just love it. Teaching a child to cook good food makes you a great parent. To take them to a fast food restaurant and not teach them to cook is almost child abuse. Many mothers and their children are blind to the problem. Health care providers must set an example, teach the parents and children and set a good example. People are shopping for quantity and not quality because I don't think they know the difference. Health education in the schools is poor.

A pediatrician walked with me through Wal-Mart, Myers, Kroger's and some other food markets and I agree that healthy fast food, when properly selected, purchased in larger quantities and prepared properly is clearly cheaper than the alternative. I wish we would have a federal law telling us what is wholesome food with a green, yellow or red light. Whole Foods labels its food with the aggregate nutrient density index (ANDI Score), invented by pediatrician Dr. Joel Fuhrman. I think that's great. But I think a green, yellow and red light would be simpler.

We are slowly killing ourselves. It is better not try to micro-manage other people's diets, said the director of an interfaith organization. Dead wrong! It's a public health problem, as Dr. Lustig and many others are recognizing.

The Wic program, a nutrition program for very young children, does have some restrictions on what type of food they can buy with it. It needs to be put across the rest of the food stamp programs. President Obama, please step up to bat. Trying to restrict food choices that are killing us probably will start a food fight. The trouble is some counties in Texas have 40% of the people on food stamps. There is a lot of politics involved. But we are paying the taxes and should have some say.

We need to pass some public health laws, with restrictions on trans fats, fat and sugar content.

The Master Disease of Our Time: Sugar Addiction

THE GREEKS SPOKE ABOUT THE mythological giant, Anteus, who became stronger whenever he touched his mother, the earth. He was conquered by Hercules when he held him off the ground.

Twenty-five hundred years ago later, we have been lifted off the earth by the modern industrial complex. We have been held captive by the power of the industrial complex and the government. It's a world of thousands of processed food items made in a plant, along with their accompanying hormones, pesticides, herbicides and genetically altered food that is killing us.

Dr. Norman Cleve, who had been the chief medical officer of a battleship in WWII, was the first to propose that taking off the germ and the bran resulted in a sugary product that caused most of Western diseases. He set out the concept that most Western diseases were caused by consuming refined carbohydrate foods.

He felt the fundamental problem lies in the fact that Westerners had a profound change in their diet in a very short period of time, which did not allow for evolutionary adaptation. Dr. D. P. Burkett from England, also way ahead of his time, agreed with that. Dr. Robert Lustig also agrees. The mass incrimination of sugar and white flour as the cause of a lot of Western diseases was first advanced by Dr. Cleve in 1956.

Dr. Cleve used the term "the saccharine disease" and published that book in 1956, so I think we may need to give them the original credit for this concept.

He also stresses the term "simplicity," reminding us that the biggest advances in humanity have been simple. He called saccharine a refined carbohydrate in that it caused a carbohydrate disease.

No distinction between the twins, glucose and fructose, and especially the evil twin fructose, was made because the science had not advanced far enough. The metabolism of fructose was likely not known at that time. Let's face it, the chemical formula for **glucose** and fructose is the same, fructose is just an isomer of glucose. Another simple explanation: High fructose corn syrup had not been invented yet either.

Dr. Cleve brings up Charles Darwin's law of adaptation. He states that there hasn't been enough time in terms of evolution for our bodies to adapt to this onslaught of new processed food.

Both Dr. Cleve and Dr. Yudkin thought that sugar was the cause of the majority of Western diseases. Dr. Cleve thought that removing fiber exposed the carbohydrates' endosperm, causing constipation, varicose veins, diverticulitis, cancer of the colon, dental disease, type 2 diabetes, obesity, vascular disease, heart attacks and strokes.

Dr. Cleve also spoke about change in our intestines, and how 500 different bacteria and viruses living there can result in a significant amount of disease.

We know of Dr. Ansell Keys entering the picture in the '50s and the studies he did in the Mediterranean area. He proposed that fat causes chronic Western diseases and eventually Dr. Cleve and Dr. Yudkin were thrown under the bus for 30 years.

But now we have defined fructose, and its metabolic effects on the liver, as a cause of Western diet-induced diseases. The real evil twin fructose has been discovered and we now know what he looks like in spite of having the same chemical configuration as glucose, $C_6H_{12}O_6$, but the atoms are arranged differently.

Sugar and the Brain

OUR ANCESTORS, HUMAN AND ANIMAL, ate fruit with fructose only a few months a year. In addition, the foods they consumed had more fiber than those we consume today.

Fructose is the weakest of all natural sugars. Fructose is low on the glycemic index because it does not stimulate insulin production.

Diabetes has profound effects on the brain because of sugar metabolism. The data regarding diabetes, dementia and Alzheimer's disease is profound. Diabetics also have a powerful risk of cognitive decline and dementia. Avoiding diabetes, especially poor control, is critical. I work a lot with the diabetic doctors, PAs and nurse practitioners who say diabetic patients have only a 50% compliance rate, so you can imagine what the sugars are doing to their body: amputations, heart attacks, strokes, dementia, vascular disease, autoimmune disease and cancer and many other illnesses, including blindness.

A more recent study recently proved a direct link between the rate of cognitive decline and increased levels of HBA 1C.

The combination of sugar and protein in the blood forms a nasty chemical combination called advanced glycation end products (AGE's). Advanced glycation products cause protein in fiber to become misshapen and inflexible. Just look at the type 2 diabetic and a smoker and the older person, those are the visible effects of advanced glycation products. You can predict the aging process in the body by obtaining a blood marker, advanced glycation product and HbA1c.

High fructose corn syrup increases the rate of glycation and formation of AGEs 10 times. You can see the problem. That is a huge statistic.

When protein becomes glycated, it binds to sugar, causes cross protein links, which gum up our vasculature, nerves, brain, eyes, organs, skin, etc. This causes free radicals, oxidation and the rotting and frying of our brain. The best way to reduce AGE's formation is proper eating and avoiding the evil twin, fructose.

The bottom line is you want to reduce oxidative stress and the action of free radicals from harming your brain and reduce your aggregated glycation end products.

Avoiding fructose is number one and also glucose because it causes obesity.

Evil Twin Detox

IF YOU WANT TO RECLAIM your health, control your future, look and feel great, then I recommend standing in front of the mirror and visualizing what you want to look like in six months. Do it at least once a week. It can be motivating and stimulating. Create a plan and follow through.

Create a mantra, a few words that you say out loud at least twice a day that will motivate you. For example," I want to get rid of my type 2 diabetes in six months,"" I'm doing this for my family,"" I want to look strong and fit."

To reduce the power of glucose and fructose, it is best to go through about 10 to 14 days of detox, a period where you are much stricter in your consumption of sugar, glucose and fructose than you normally need to be. I would even give up alcohol for two weeks because it is a sugar. This will reduce your fructose enzymes in the liver and stabilize the addictive power of sugar on the brain.

Nutrient-dense foods, through something called nutrigenomics, have acquired genes that affect food metabolism through epigenetics, in other words have the ability to repair your sick genes. Food is information. I was recently at a conference and an addiction specialist told me, you can detox from sugar or narcotics many times in 1 week.

Your body would reset metabolic food chains and begin the healing of your body. Food is medicine.

Dr. Richard Johnson recommends a two-week detox and I agree with that. This will repair the damage done by high fructose diet. This will repair the gut, because, after all, fructose, corn syrup for example, punches holes in your intestine, allowing undigested food to get into the bloodstream, causing immune reactions, which make you sick. The detox will quickly repair the fructose enzymes in your liver, which lead to insulin resistance, leptin resistance and fatty liver.

In the long run you would do fine by simply reducing your fructose intake by 30 to 50%, but in the short term, we want to radically change your metabolism as well as educate you as to what the fructose content is in many different foods. Be sure to use the tables of fructose content of foods and restaurants in this book; they are also illustrated in Dr. Richard Johnson's "A Sugar Fix."

Fructose Free for Two Weeks

WE NEED TO REDUCE THE number of fructose enzymes. We don't eliminate all fructose, because some vegetables and other foods contain a small amount, which is of no consequence to you. Remember, usually you can consume up to 35 grams of fructose a day and be very healthy. The trouble is we are consuming 66 grams a day.

There is no need to count calories. Included is a list of foods that you can eat in the first two-week period and you will notice that they contain less than 1 gram of sugar in a standard serving, and the majority of them have less than 0.5 grams of fructose sugar.

High Fructose Foods

HIGH FRUCTOSE FOODS INCLUDE CANDY, cookies, cakes, pies, and other baked goods, fruit, fruit juice and other beverages that contain fruit, honey, sports drinks, soda and other soft drinks. You must become very conscious as to what the fructose content of food is and start reading labels. Especially avoid high fructose corn syrup, but then again all fructose is dangerous.

There are many variations of the terms sucrose or table sugar: beet sugar, brown sugar, cane sugar, corn sweetener, corn syrup, maple syrup, glasses, raw sugar, sucrose, table sugar, etc.

Eliminating food from your diet for two weeks means you may be missing some important nutrients. For this reason, I recommend taking some supplements for a few weeks: a multivitamin with minerals, plus 50 mg of vitamin C.

Consider avoiding restaurants and take-out food during the fructose free phase, because it's hard to be certain if the food you're ordering contains sugar or high fructose corn syrup. You should drink five cups of water per day. If you need to drink alcohol, consume only one glass of wine a day or less.

The Problem with Fruit

REMEMBER, FRUIT HAS FRUCTOSE IN it and does not metabolize any differently, to my dismay. Then again, it has a lot of fiber with it and after the first two-week period, I think it is reasonable to eat two or three servings a day if your health is improving. If you have metabolic syndrome or type 2 diabetes, you probably will correct that very quickly if you're really watching your fructose.

A Short Review

SUGAR MAY BE BAD, BUT the sweetener called fructose is far more deadly.

A 2009 study from the University of California, Davis, and additional scientific studies confirm that consuming high fructose corn syrup is the fastest way to trash your health. It is now known, without a doubt, that sugar in food, in all its myriad forms, is taking a devastating toll.

Fructose in any form, including high fructose corn syrup and crystalline fructose, is the worst of the worst. Fructose, a cheap sweetener usually derived from corn, is used in thousands of food products and soft drinks. Excessive fructose consumption can cause metabolic damage and trigger the early stages of diabetes and heart disease.

Dr. Richard Johnson does a fabulous job of comprehensively reviewing this important topic in his new book, "The Fat Switch." Fructose consumption leads to insulin resistance, obesity, elevated blood pressure, elevated triglycerides and elevated LDL, depletion of vitamins and minerals, cardiovascular disease, liver disease, fatty liver, cancer, arthritis and even gout.

A Calorie in is Not a Calorie out!

GLUCOSE IS A FORM OF energy you were designed to run on. Every cell in your body, every area and in fact every little thing on earth uses glucose for energy.

If you receive fructose only from vegetables and fruits as most people did a century ago, you would consume about 15 grams per day, a far cry from the 73 grams per day the typical adolescent consumes from sweetened drinks. In vegetables and fruits, fructose is mixed with fiber, vitamins, minerals, enzymes and beneficial phyto-nutrients, all of which moderate any negative metabolic effects.

It isn't the fructose itself that is bad; it's the massive dose most people consume that makes it dangerous.

Your body metabolizes fructose in a much different way than glucose. The entire burden of metabolizing fructose falls on your liver. People are consuming fructose in enormous quantities, which has made the negative effects much more profound. Today, 55% of sweeteners used in food and beverage manufacturing are made from corn, and the number one source of calories in America is soda, in the form of high fructose corn syrup.

Fructose Metabolism Reviewed

AFTER EATING FRUCTOSE, 100% OF the metabolic burden rests on your liver, as opposed to only 20 percent with glucose.

Every cell in your body, including your brain, utilizes glucose. By contrast, fructose is turned into free fatty acids, VLDL, very low-density LDL, triglycerides that get stored as fat. The fatty acids created during fructose metabolism accumulate as fat droplets in your liver and skeletal muscle tissues, causing insulin resistance and non-alcoholic liver disease, and insulin resistance progresses to metabolic syndrome and type 2 diabetes.

Fructose is the most lipophilic carbohydrate. In addition, fructose converts to activated glycerol, G3 P, which forms free fatty acids, resulting in triglycerides and fat. The more G3 P you have, the more fat you store. Glucose does not do this. Fructose and glucose cause our triglycerides to be high, not fat!

One hundred and twenty calories of fructose results in 40 calories being stored as fat. Consuming fructose is essentially consuming fat! The metabolism of fructose creates a long list of waste products and toxins, including large amounts of uric acid, which drives up blood pressure and causes gout.

Glucose depresses the hunger hormone ghrelin and interferes with your brains communication with leptin, resulting in overeating.

If anyone tries to tell you sugar is just glucose, they're way behind the times. The bottom line is that fructose leads to increased belly fat, insulin resistance and metabolic syndrome, not to mention a long list of chronic diseases. Eating sugar will accelerate the aging process itself.

Dump the Dairy

OF THE WORLD'S 5,400 MAMMALS, each one produces specially designed milk for its infants. Each type of milk is different when it comes to the amount of protein, carbohydrates and fat.

Why would we want to drink the milk of a cow, which contains 57 hormones, pesticides and herbicides? No other mammal drinks the milk of another mammal, except for humans.

The enzymes we need to digest the lactose in milk decrease significantly by age 4 and 70% of people are born without the ability to digest milk properly. Asians lack the enzyme to break down lactose in milk, 75% of African-Americans are also missing the enzyme. Only 50% of white people have that enzyme.

Infants need mother's milk for good health and metabolism and great brain growth. It supplies the good omega-3 fats.

Cow's milk, however, is unnecessary in the human diet. The U.S. Department of Agriculture's "My Plate" recommends three glasses of low-fat milk a day. That's just plain wrong and not good for children's health. The rate of type 1 diabetes is higher in children who drink cow's milk, and there are many allergies associated with lactose, including infections. Many people's gastrointestinal tracts do not tolerate casein, the protein in milk.

A lot of disease occurs because of that which can be completely avoided.

Without lactase, lactose remains undigested, fermenting in your intestine and causing an array of gastrointestinal symptoms that we refer to as lactose intolerance. Even if your body can break down lactose, it's still bad news, because it is converted to galactose and glucose which elevates blood sugar, causes inflammation and insulin resistance.

Casein, the protein in milk, can prove toxic and eventually lead to neurodegenerative diseases, including attention deficit disorder.

You don't need calcium from milk to keep your bones strong and ward off osteoporosis. Plants have plenty of calcium and are a better source for it. Incidentally, high animal meat protein diets will make the blood acidic, leaching calcium out of the bones in attempt to make the blood more alkaline.

Green leafy vegetables, vitamin D supplements, exercise and increased protein from vegetables are more effective ways for your body to get the calcium it needs.

There are some other reasons for not drinking milk. Milk is generally pasteurized, a heating process to kill bacteria which also kills most of the enzymes that may have made milk slightly worth drinking. It renders milk relatively useless, nutritionally speaking. Cows are generally given growth hormones, which stimulates your liver to produce insulin growth factor, which increases the rate of breast, colon and prostate cancer. These growth hormones are suspected of contributing to early puberty in children. The increase rate of cancer in both children and adults who drink a lot of milk is especially concerning.

Dr. Veerula and Dr. Fuhrman have noticed a tremendous reduction in illness, including infections, allergies, type I diabetes and cancer in their patients who don't drink milk. They say that milk is "liquid meat" and do not recommend it.

Artificial Sweeteners

ARTIFICIAL SWEETENERS ARE INCREASINGLY USED to satisfy a sweet tooth. Unfortunately, the only one I recommend is Stevia. It's a natural plant from Mexico and most people think it is quite safe. Stevia leaves are 10 to 15 times sweeter than sugar, although a problem with artificial sweeteners is it will increase your desire for other sweets.

If you are switching from sugar to artificial sweeteners, you are jumping from the frying pan into the fire. That's the opinion of many nutritionists.

Artificial sweeteners actually elevate insulin levels, because they signal to the brain that something sweet is coming even though it is not. The brain secretes hormones that do that. Artificial sweeteners can distort metabolic hormonal messages and trigger hunger, because they provide no calories; the longer this goes on, the more you will eat. Artificial sweeteners are known to cause belly fat and weight gain. Artificial sweeteners also contribute to sugar cravings and sugar addiction, because they are much sweeter than sugar. Also, artificial sweeteners are created by chemical processes that require the use of strong chemicals, which can further harm the body. If you need a sweetener, Stevia the best option, according to many nutritionists. I use nothing and have a four-pack for a belly. I will be 78 next month!

The History of Glucose and Fructose

AROUND 10,000 YEARS AGO, JUST about when we started agriculture and eventually raising cattle, a plant was discovered in New Guinea called sugarcane. It is a combination of **glucose and fructose**. All plants produce some sucrose. As a result glucose and fructose are found throughout nature, just different amounts in different plants.

Sucrose is a disaccharide, a combination of 50% each. Lactose is a combination of galactose and glucose. All sugars are sweet, but glucose is 50 to 60% as sweet as fructose. Honey is much sweeter and is 70% fructose. High fructose corn syrup is 55% fructose, 42% glucose. It's a lot sweeter and cheaper.

We are hardwired to seek sugar based on evolution. A survival mechanism. Nature has designed pleasure as a survival mechanism and uses food and sex to do it.

Fruit was probably not cultivated until around 6,000 years ago. Of course the main sugar in fruit is fructose. It is also metabolized in the liver just like the fructose from sucrose.

Our ancestors probably ate 15 to 20 grams of fructose a day. A typical American probably consumes 70-80 grams a day now. Twenty percent of Americans consume 15 to 20% of their diet that way.

Sugarcane spread to Australia, India, Persia and Europe and eventually to Spain and Crete. It was first introduced in England around the year of 1000. Christopher Columbus brought sugarcane to Haiti and the Dominican Republic on his second voyage to the New World in 1493. Further, a lot of sugar was imported back to Europe. It started the candy revolution. The Germans in 1747 found that sugar beets were also good source of sugar. Candy bars were sold throughout the 19th century.

Frankly, obesity is probably worse than the plague ever was. The suffering last longer and is now worldwide.

Liquid White Gold

COCA-COLA WAS DISCOVERED IN A pharmacy in Atlanta in 1886 and started a revolution in sugary products. In 1968, it was discovered that if you took an enzyme called glucose isomerase, you could make corn syrup a lot sweeter and cheaper because the government was supporting the price of corn. In 1971 the Japanese discovered a way of converting the sugar in corn syrup to fructose and the rest is history.

Fructose increases the shelf life of processed foods, makes food cheaper and sweeter, increases the rate of sugar joining up with proteins in the blood, which increases the rate of aging and is the cause of a lot of diseases including dementia. It also affects the brain, increasing appetite.

In the 1950s, '60s and '70s, Dr. Cleve and Dr. Yudkin proposed the sugar theory of disease, but they were thrown under the bus for 30 years by the "fat theory" as the cause of obesity and chronic disease. The latter is being disproven at this time. Be sure to read Dr. Richard Johnson's "Sugar Fix" and "Fat Change," and Dr. Richard Lustig's "Fat Chance."

Our genetic structure has changed very little in the last hundred thousand years. Food is information, and our bodies are revolting against the new foods, resulting in chronic diseases.

Fructose: The Lipinator

ARE WE THE MOST OBESE nation on earth because of lack of will-power? Other nations think so, but I don't agree. For one thing, many other nations are also becoming overweight. Look at Mexico, which just passed the United States to become the most obese nation on earth. Vietnam and South Korea are running high rates of obesity and type 2 diabetes.

We are programmed through evolution to store **energy** as a survival mechanism; nature even attached pleasure to it. Food has overpowered us, we don't know how to cook, glucose and fructose are found throughout our many thousands of processed food items in the food markets. Most are creations of industrial, rather than natural, plants.

Fructose is sweeter than glucose, more tasty, and it offers your brain more reward, turning off the appetite suppressants leptin and ghrelin from your stomach. This means that we might sit down and eat a dozen donuts or a bag of chips. We also know now that fructose depletes your liver of energy, ATP, causes fatty liver and introduces very low density LDL, which is the cause of many health problems.

Eating a high-fat diet can certainly make you fatter if that's a problem to begin with, but the effects of fructose are much more severe.

Fructose fails to satisfy our hunger because it causes leptin resistance, which fails to regulate our fat deposits. We now know that fat is a gland: It is very active producing hormones, enzymes, cytokines, leptin, etc.

Eating a fructose-rich diet disrupts our metabolism, causing changes in our fat cells. Eating a high fructose diet is one of many ways to increase oxidative stress, a metabolic process related to many diseases. Fructose is 10 times more effective at creating sugar protein products called AGEs, advanced glycation products, which inflame our bodies. Oxidative free radicals are the product of oxygen in sugar metabolism, which is accentuated with fructose metabolism.

Chronic fructose consumption causes insulin resistance, which ends up increasing blood sugar. The sugar attaches to proteins in the blood, resulting in disease and the aging process.

Fructose metabolism is a huge cause of nonalcoholic fatty liver disease, cryptogenic cirrhosis, which is the biggest cause of liver transplants. This will be a huge cost to the nation in the future.

The International Fat Epidemic

SURVIVAL OF THE FATTEST IS a new paradigm.

There are 1½ billion obese people in the world, and 100 million dying yearly as a result of the complications of heart disease, stroke, type 2 diabetes, cancer, autoimmune diseases and numerous other illnesses. All of this is produced by what's on our spoons and forks and the sugary drinks we consume.

There is an evolutionary fight between our genetic structure and the genes of our food. There has not been enough time over the course of evolution to change our genetic structure to mitigate the threats to our health. It's an equal opportunity employer.

It's occurring throughout the world now. It used to be just the Western societies, but it is spreading like the plague throughout Asia, South Vietnam, South Korea, the Middle East, Europe, the Persian Gulf and especially many of the isolated islands of the Pacific. On one Pacific island, Natur, 95% of the people are obese. It's happening in Africa where they used to eat mainly vegetables and had none of these problems. Some groups are affected more than others based on education, race, poverty and sedentary lifestyle.

The great pandemics of history were the" Black Death plague" of the 14th century that killed 45 million people. It was caused by bacteria, yersinia pestis. It killed quickly, in a matter of days.

The Spanish flu of 1918 was also very deadly. It killed 40 million people from a virus within weeks.

The ongoing epidemic we are having from AIDS has been shown to be caused by a virus from mammals in Africa. It's killed about 25 million people so far and 100 million may be infected. The new drugs are helping a great deal.

It is the opinion of Dr. Richard Johnson that the greatest epidemic of all is obesity and its secondary diseases, which have killed so many people over the decades. It's my opinion that obesity will have killed 200 million people a year in another 10 to 15 years and maybe more. It will kill more people than all the other illnesses and epidemics combined. The difference though is the present epidemic can be stopped, prevented and cured.

The *Wall Street Journal* recently carried a great exposé on the obesity and diabetic problem across the world but especially in the Persian Gulf countries. It is caused by lack of exercise, the sugary food and a sedentary lifestyle. Likewise, the *New York Times* ran an expose describing the great increase in obesity surgery on children in the Persian Gulf countries. There wasn't much talk in either article on the food they were eating. Let's face it: If parents didn't feed children sugary foods, the epidemics wouldn't exist. Parents are having the same problem and that complicates matters tremendously. Education is the key.

Dr. James Neal proposed the "Thrifty Gene" hypothesis in 1961. He suggested that the rise in obesity and diabetes observed throughout the world today was due to the genes that we acquired in the past. He points out that the animals and insects had the ability to store fat, and survived because of it. Evolution selected them to be the parents of the future.

The story of hibernation of different living creatures tells the real story. Some frogs can survive five years without eating. Whales don't eat while swimming 5,000 kilometers to their place of reproduction in Mexico. The hummingbird stores up to 40% fat in one day from eating sugar. Its liver literally turns white.

Dr. Neil suggests that during periods of famine, those individuals who carried the gene that would favor the greatest accumulation of fat would be more likely to survive. Asians, African-Americans, people in the Persian Gulf and some Americans carry more of these genes and you can see **the** results if they eat the wrong food. If they eat mainly a plant diet, they are perfectly healthy and thin.

So eating too much and lack of exercise is not the total answer, it's what **you are** eating.

Some people are just more prone to become overweight if they eat the wrong food. Sugar, especially fructose and saturated fats including polyunsaturated omega-6s, lead to obesity.

Living things, animals, amphibians, insects, etc. even develop insulin resistance when getting ready for hibernation. But when they are done hibernating, the switch is turned off and they get back to their normal weight, within .5%, quickly.

But we humans don't. Some say it's a rheostat and not a switch, we've lost control of the mechanism.

Dr. Richard Johnson feels its loss of the uric acid enzyme, uricase, that's supposed to destroy uric acid and clear it out of the body through the kidneys that is the problem. That was lost thousands of years ago through the process of evolution. Uric acid increases fat deposits, and the only people who didn't have this enzyme lived and were selected throughout evolution for survival. He feels the same thing happened with the ability to make vitamin C. Vitamin C reduces fat deposits, and evolution favored those who didn't have the vitamin C gene. In other words this double knockout of this uricase enzyme and loss of vitamin C increased our propensity to keep the fat switch on. It was a survival mechanism.

Weight is Tightly Controlled in Nature

THE EMPEROR PENGUIN WILL NOT eat for six months while the male incubates the egg lying on his feet. He is totally dependent on the fat stored in his abdomen. He has developed insulin resistance. He stored up the fat throughout the summer and is dependent on his fat switch.

The increase in fat is scheduled and regulated by nature. Unfortunately that is not the case in humans. Most wild animals by nature have become periodically obese by evolutionary design. The ones that couldn't do it died out. Animals will switch from fat accumulation, phase 2 of fat burning, on genetic demand. It's highly regulated.

What happened to us? Being fat had a survival advantage in evolution.

Most animals store fat very similar to us. Subcutaneous, liver, bowel, neck, back, buttocks, and abdomen etc., although a recent article indicated that hibernating bears, the grizzly bear specifically, did not store the fat in its organs but under the skin. Interesting. I bet he doesn't have insulin resistance. Seals can weigh up to 3,000 pounds and then fast up to 60 days while swimming to another reproductive site. Humans can go without eating for only about a month.

In hibernation, animals decrease their metabolic rate, reduce their temperature and reduce up to 90% of their usual energy needs. Hibernation is a powerful mechanism of decreasing energy needs. The basic metabolic rate goes way down. You can see how important our basic metabolic rate is when you look at its effect on fat metabolism and energy needs.

Sugar, especially fructose, is accompanied by hypertension, arterial disease, vascular disease, heart attacks, strokes, and cancer and is killing us.

The French physician Etienne Lancereaux, 1829-1891, separated type 1 diabetes, no insulin, from type 2 diabetes, too much insulin. Type 1 patients are lean and type 2 are overweight. But now many advanced type 2 diabetics become lean because they lose the ability to make insulin, their pancreas is dying out and now they have both diseases and soon will be on dialysis, have visual loss, nerve loss, amputations, memory loss etc.? Prevention is the key.

Metabolic syndrome was first described in 1920 and then popularized by Dr. Gerald Raven in the 1980s. Twenty-five percent of people in the United States have metabolic syndrome. That includes hypertension, and a waistline greater than 40 inches for males and 35 inches for females as well as high triglycerides, greater than 150, high LDL, low HDL and a fasting blood sugar greater than 110. If you have two or three of these, you have metabolic syndrome. Probably 100 to 250 million people in the United States have it. It's an epidemic here and across the world.

Insulin resistance accompanies the fat storage of hibernation and is in the crosshairs of metabolic syndrome and our obesity story. Animals preparing for food storage turn on the fats, which cause insulin resistance.

The squirrels, penguins, whales, fish, birds, they all do it. The hummingbird will run blood sugars up to 700; the liver becomes white from eating nectar, high fructose sugar, in one day.

Metabolic syndrome should be called the fat storage syndrome. That's why I wrote my last book called "The Golden Opportunity" to encourage providers to diagnose this increasing medical problem very early. I recommend health risk assessment and blood testing starting as a young child and then possibly we might avoid most of this plague.

Insulin resistance is a survival factor in animals, but it's killing us because we have lost the uricase enzyme and the ability to make vitamin C and they control the fat switch in the mitochondria, according to Dr. Richard Johnson, and I agree with that after reviewing the relevant medical literature.

Animals develop metabolic syndrome to survive. But food is plentiful for us and we don't need it. Very little evolutionary selection will occur among humans in the future because we're dying generally beyond the reproductive age and nature will not get panicked about it. But we are leading sickly lives, losing our memory and dying young of chronic diseases. Very little evolutionary selection will occur. Most people will be through the reproductive years before they die.

Obesity is not from gluttony and idleness, but because we've activated the same switch all animals use to increase fat stores. Industry is, of course, looking for the pill to affect the fat switch. Good luck fighting the survival mechanism of Mother Nature. I'd rather teach you how to eat correctly.

The cause of obesity is that we are eating too much and exercising too little, right? Culture, economics and behavior support that. Eating too much, because of fast food, cheap food, allows us to ingest massive amounts of calories. All-you-can-eat buffets, sugary drinks, high fructose corn syrup and lack of exercise on top of that.

The average child is exposed to 40,000 food advertisements a year, 72% for fast food.

Animals have a set point, we don't. Probably because we lack the ability to throw the fat switch off. The lack of uricase enzyme acquired in evolution is largely responsible.

Obesity is generally measured by the BMI, body mass index: Weight/kilogram divided by height in meters squared, 20-25 is normal, 25-30 is overweight, greater than 35 is obese, greater than 42 was morbidly obese.

The Obese are on Fire

THE FRUCTOSE PRESENT IN FRUITS, vegetables and high fructose drinks is part of the driver of our obesity epidemic, although just plain sugar, which is 50% fructose, probably is the main person at the wheel.

Let's face it; carrot cake has 50 grams of fructose.

One in five people in the Persian Gulf has type 2 diabetes, while 40% are obese, higher than in the United States. I bet you 70% or higher have "diabesity," the path to type 2 diabetes. Saudi Arabia and Kuwait are leading the way and are surrounded by countries that are also being invaded by this epidemic.

Thirty-five million people in the Middle East and North Africa have type 2 diabetes -- 11% of the world has now come down with the disease. The situation is predicted to become much worse. It is predicted to grow to 68 million in the Middle East by 2035. Sub Sahara Africa is having great increases at this time.

I found out recently that the famous clinic "Lifestyle Institute in Arizona", which had reversed type 2 diabetes over a three week period for 30 years, has closed according to an operator I spoke to. They did follow-up studies and found very poor compliance in their former patients. Due to these poor long-term results, they decided to close. This has put an arrow through my heart, but it will not stop me and I will just redouble my efforts. After all, I am a doctor.

The good news is that this plague can be prevented, stopped and reversed. Let's get to work. Ninety percent of type 2 diabetes can be stopped, reversed and prevented over just four to eight weeks. But, we need good follow up to make sure that we are inducing a permanent change. Low compliance rates are not going to work. Then again, most people can indeed be cured the majority of the time.

Dr. Mehmet Oz says," inflammation is the rusting of your arteries." Inflammation is a fire where you can't see the flames. It remains hidden for many years until you run some tests, and then it might be too late.

The Good Fats

YES, WE HAVE SOME GOOD fats, and they are essential for our existence.

They have been with us since the beginning of time. They are called essential fatty acids, have to be consumed as food, and we could not live without them.

Millions of years ago before we developed a circulatory system, we used fatty acids as communicators, like the internet; they were then and still are today our basic communicating system between our 70 trillion cells. They are rapidly made and destroyed making them difficult to study. They were first identified in the prostate gland, which is why you hear the term prostaglandins; you have to collect thousands of animal prostate glands just to have a few for study.

The essential fats omega-3 and omega-6 are converted through enzymatic processes to various other fatty acids like EPA, DHA and the anti-inflammatories and the pro-inflammatory AA arachnodinic acid, prostaglandins, thromboxane and leukotrines. Our ancient ancestors ate a ratio of omega-3 versus omega-6 of about 2:3. We are now eating omega-6s 20/1 over omega-3s. We are indeed inflamed. We are on fire. That's why we see so much advanced disease, heart disease, strokes, cancer, autoimmune disease, dementia and more.

The pro-inflammatory fatty acids are found in animal products, genetically modified corn, high fructose corn syrup and cattle from concentrated animal feeding organizations as well as pond-raised fish. When eating or shopping out, always ask - where did this beef or fish come from? That's why it is important to eat organic raised beef, lamb pork and fish.

Things got a lot more interesting though when Dr. Bang and Dr. Dyerberg from Denmark went to Greenland and studied the Eskimos. At that time there was a lot of nasty disease and diabetes in Denmark, but they had heard that the Eskimos were eating a very high-fat diet but had little evidence of heart attacks, strokes and cancer. This work was done in the 1960s and 1970s.

The Eskimos were eating at 50% fat diet of blubber from seals and whales and had little evidence of heart disease, vascular disease and diabetes.

In 2003 we switched from a low-fat regimen to high-fat diet. The Atkins diet became the rage. We followed the advice of Dr. Ansell Keys for 30 years and become sicker every year. About 50% of people now have diabesity and we are heading even higher.

The first of omega-3s, alphlinoleic acid or ALA, is the parent of these fatty acids. They are found mainly in the leaves of plants and other green parts of the plants. They are associated with the photosynthetic process of plants. Yes, plants have some fat in them; even though it is not very much per plant, it is the most prevalent essential fatty acid in the universe considering the pure volume of plant structures.

One glycerol and three fatty acids make one triglyceride, your fat molecule.

DHA, Docosahexaenoic acid, is a child of alpha-linonic acid. DHA is used by humans and animals for vision, thinking, nerve conduction and is a fast moving fatty acid. It is related to the structure of the fatty acid. These essential fatty acids move very quickly and have a short lifespan. DHEA is the quick-change artist. Your brain is full of DHEA.

Alpha-linonic acid is found in the chloroplasts of plants, the green part. It is the most abundant fat on earth. DHA and EPA accumulate in animals because they eat the plants. Deficiencies of EPA, DHA, have resulted in a host of human illnesses including vascular disease; type 2 diabetes, cancer, dementia, etc.

DHA needs to be in our eyes, brain, heart and all other tissues. That's why ocean fish and some omega-3 supplements, like EPA, ALA and DHA have value.

DHA was not the first of omega-3s discovered; that was EPA-eicosopentic acid. It has 20 carbon atoms, eikosi means 20 in Greek.

These were discovered by the two Danish physicians, Dr. Bang and Dr. Dyerberg who studied the Eskimos in Greenland in the 1970s. They studied the Eskimos and their blood with gas-liquid-chromatography, a fairly new invention.

They published a paper in the journal *Lancet* suggesting that the explanation for the Eskimos' longevity and lack of disease was the consumption of large amounts of poly-unsaturated fat. They eventually went to Minnesota to run further studies on the Eskimo blood in the laboratory of Dr. Mark Holman, the world's fat expert at that time.

He found the Eskimos had a high concentration of the good cholesterol, HDL, the one that cleans out your arteries, low levels of bad cholesterol LDL, and even lower levels of very low-density LDL or bad cholesterol. Gas chromatography was needed to differentiate the different fats. What I'm saying is that all fat is not the same. Essential fatty acids, unsaturated fats and some polyunsaturated fats can be good for you; saturated, or hydroge-nated, fats are killers. They were separated apart by their boiling points and molecular weight.

The omegas got their name from Dr. Mark Holman.

It's my opinion the reason the Eskimos didn't develop these chronic diseases is related to the critical essential fatty acids they were consuming as well as their low consumption of the evil twin, fructose, and it's malignant brother, glucose.

Dr. Holman wrote in 1964, "the concept of a balanced diet must include a ratio of several essential fat asses including mono-unsaturated, unsaturated, Omega threes etc." The U.S. Depart-ment of Agriculture doesn't mention that in the most recent dietary recommendations. Fat was vilified in the 1960s, vegeta-ble oil was vilified in the 1980s, trans fats in the 1990s and look at the result. The public is so confused that they still don't know what they should take most of the time, and, if they do, they don't know why they're taking it.

Dr. Ralph Holman has studied fats most of his professional life. Interestingly enough Dr. Ansell Keys, the enemy of fat, was also from Minnesota. He had a strong personality and few were willing to question his theory. But then again this was before a lot of the different fats were understood, according to a lot of scien-tists, although he never adjusted his opinion after new informa-tion become available.

The point is that all fats are not alike.

People had less heart disease during and after World War II and they were eating less meat, butter, cheese, and eggs. That has been well studied. When the above foods returned, people got sick again. Dr. Bang and Dr. Dyerberg did not know that they had upset the old model of Ansell Keys.

The omega-6s, which are pro-inflammatory, promotes blood clotting, vasoconstriction, pain, cell division, depression, decreased effectiveness of the immune system and increased memory loss.

So now we know some of the history of essential fatty acids. As a reminder, they should be in a proper ratio of 1 to 1, 2 to 2 or 3 to 2, not 20 to 1.

In 2005, the Studer Group studied 275,000 subjects. In the study, omega-3s were shown to reduce risk factors by 32% and mortality by 23%. That is a huge statistic. What you eat and drink has a tremendous effect on your health.

More than 70 clinical trials have demonstrated the consistent glycemic lowering effect of fish oil supplements. Some studies have shown a triglyceride reducing effect as high as 79% compared to controls. Dr. Joe C.Maroon's book "Fish Oil" describes this in detail.

The main cause of vascular disease is inflammation. We have 300,000 miles of microvasculature, which is pretty amazing when you think about it. Vascular disease is the main cause of death globally, although cancer may surpass that statistic this year.

The main cause of vascular disease is turning on the fat switch; it's the twin's glucose and fructose, especially the latter – it's not cholesterol and some fats are even good.

The infiltration of our organs, including the liver, pancreas, and even our heart, by fat produced by the metabolism of fructose is the real Lex Luther, according to Dr. Robert Lustig.

All of this causes inflammation throughout our body, which means many people throughout the world are on fire. You don't see the flames because they are hidden in their body, but the results will show up sometime, in some very quickly.

When getting your blood work done, it is important to differentiate between LDL and Vldl. The very low-density LDL has such small molecules it takes a special test to diagnose them; one test is called "NMR" test and is not ordered routinely, so you have to ask for it. That is very important, since your life is at stake.

How do you put omega-3s back into your diet?

1) Consume oils that have a healthy balance of omega 3 and omega 6. Consume more flaxseed, walnuts, canola and soybean oils. Olive oil is good but limit it to 1 tablespoon daily, since, after all, it's 100% fat.

2) Eat lots of fruits and vegetables. Remember all plants contain some alpha-linolenic acid, the good fat.

3) Eat ocean-raised fish. Most fish today is raised on a farm and should be avoided. It is full of omega-6x versus ocean fish, which has many omega-3s.

4) Include some source of omega-3 in every meal. Add some nuts to your salads and you'll be doing it.

5) Avoid hydrogenated oils. They are full of trans fats and are not good for you.

6) Choose free-range chicken. Avoid animal products from organized farming organizations. They eat bad fats and you in turn will eat a lot of omega-6s. Likewise, when fish are fed corn.

7) Cut down on saturated fats. Fats are not as much a concern as fructose but if you're overweight, they will become a problem.

8) Check your BMI and maintain a healthy weight. I encourage you to weigh yourself every day, make a mental picture of what you want like to look at in three months and celebrate small gains.

CHO-Carbohydrate Metabolism

A CARBOHYDRATE IS A COMPLEX sugar compound and has to be broken apart to be metabolized. Some compounds have a lot of fiber, especially resisted starch. About 25% of the calories may be lost in metabolism because of the fiber and that's the good news. So it's not calories in and calories out.

But when carbohydrates are metabolized, the part that is absorbed is glucose and fructose. And they are used up, stored or changed to fat.

In 1750, we consumed 4 pounds of sugar yearly, in 1850, 20 pounds yearly, in 1994, 120 pounds, in 1990, it was 160 pounds. Let's face it, now it's probably around 200 pounds. This is well described in the book of Nora T. Gedgaudas in "Primal body, primal mind."

This estimate does not include all the hidden sources of sugar found in our thousands of manufactured foods. This doesn't even count high fructose corn syrup, which has been estimated to be about 80 pounds per year in the American diet. This huge increase can cause severe metabolic damage to us.

Our bodies are revolting in response to this onslaught on our genetic history.

Under the statistics, include the amount of sugar in our diets from other sources like carbohydrates, starches, cereals, breads, pastas, grains, potatoes and other types of sugar.

This is insanity.

Fruit, more than 2-3 pieces unfortunately is not a health food either, as fructose is the main sugar and is different from the fruits of millions of years ago. They have been seriously genetically modified to be sweeter as that is what sells. The industry knows the limits of our sweet tooth. Sugar sells, the sweeter it is the better it sells.

Sugar is both a carbohydrate and eventually a fat. That is what Dr. Robert Lustig emphasizes. The sugar stimulates an increase in insulin. Which is an anabolic hormone and causes weight increase.

Sugar and carbohydrates stimulate insulin, the anabolic fat storage hormone, which by process of glycation combines protein and sugar forming advanced glycation end product, AGE's, which are the cause of a lot of diseases.

Bread, pastas, cereals, potatoes, fried food, desserts, alcohol and unfortunately much of the fruit we eat have a great deal of fructose and you must be aware of that.

We accept blood glucose levels of 85-100, but our ancestors were averaging probably 70-85 levels.

Longevity studies are revealing 70-85 is a lot healthier if you don't develop hypoglycemia. We are not used to those levels so that might happen. Our ancestors probably had no problem with that.

The rule of thumb is that the lower your HBA 1C is, the longer you will live. It's a marker of aging.

The less sugar you eat, the better will be your health. A bagel contains 6 teaspoon full of glucose, I admit I ate a dozen once after a stressful day. Remember the fructose will not turn your appetite off like glucose might.

Cereals and potatoes can raise blood sugar levels faster than a candy bar.

Glucose in the bloodstream, especially fructose, oxidize and release free radicals, creating advanced glycation end products (AGE's) and secondary inflammation throughout the body.

Keytones from fats are more stable and don't raise the blood sugar or insulin level and can supply fuel for the brain. They also cause bad breath. Our red blood cells need oxygen and sugar to function in all the stages of our life. They create the energy molecule ATP.

Aging is now being understood by people who research longevity as essentially a gradual process of glycation. Chronic disease is associated with aging and certain forms of dementia. You see a lot more dementia in type II diabetics.

Whenever glucose is not immediately used for the acute activities of life, physical activity for example, and maintaining the metabolism of our body, is converted to glycogen. This stored glycogen in the liver and muscles will be converted to fat.

Glucagon, epinephrine, norepinephrine, cortisone and growth hormone also regulate blood sugar. Blood sugar lowering is a trivial sideline for insulin, contrary to what most people know about it.

Nature never would've made us totally dependent on just one mechanism of blood sugar control, it's too important.

We need a steady flow of fuel. Our bodies with our consumption of fructose are basically on fire. We need to feed directly, consistently and that's why we are creating the fuel. We have adapted our bodies to do this.

Contrary to most knowledge, alcoholics have issues with sugar addiction. Alcoholics are dependent and seek out fast sources of sugar, like alcohol, which is rapidly absorbed and metabolized in the liver, unfortunately, some of it goes to the brain. Once an alcoholic always an alcoholic. It's a quick sugar fix. We need to eat daily.

I know a couple people who had a problem with alcohol, but only gained a little bit of weight, largely because of poor nutrition and lack of exercise; once they stopped consuming alcohol, they gained a lot of weight. They exploded with their sugar addiction. I'm concerned about their livers. First alcohol and its sugars causing fatty liver and now all the fructose through the consumption of sugary foods is doing a double whammy to their liver.

The real problem is addiction to glucose and fructose.

Go to any AAA meeting and what are they serving? Donuts and cookies, which serve to further feed the addiction.

Nora T. Gedgaudas calls them "carbovores." I call them respectfully "carboholics."

Turning the body more in the direction of low sugar and good fats is the answer.

Nature would never have held us only dependent on sugar.

Our primal ancestors would never have made it only on a sugar diet.

Most people adapted to a state of carbohydrate and sugar metabolism and look at the result-obesity and chronic disease. Most people manage their blood sugar levels by eating sugary foods all day long.

They need to stoke the fire that's occurring in their body.

Dietary fat, in the absence of carbohydrate, is like putting a nice big log on the fire. It keeps going for long time and reduces the ups and downs. Fat does not raise blood sugar quickly and only when it's used up in energy metabolism.

Metabolically we are having a failure to communicate with our evolutionary hormonal system. Only one percent of the pancreas is devoted to insulin secretion.

Type II diabetes is a disease of the blood sugar because of insulin resistance. That's why the level of insulin in the blood is more important even than the blood sugar level, especially in the 10 to 15 years before a diagnosis is ever made. A recent study published in the "New England Journal of Medicine 2008" stated that they were surprised to find that increased insulin use actually caused an increase in death from heart attack and stroke. It was the result of the ACCORD study. The study was actually cut short due to these alarming findings. This unfortunately continues to be the standard in diabetic care, a focus on blood sugar instead of insulin resistance. The key is the restoration of insulin sensitivity and cellular communication.

Keep It Simple

THE FOLLOWING TIPS WILL MAKE it simple for you to eat and live well:

1) Make a commitment.
2) Use a mantra – empowering words that inspire you such as -"I want to live to be hundred without disease, look good, honor my god or spirit."
3) Visualize the result daily: Make a mental picture of how you want to look and feel.
4) Educate yourself and participate in your healthcare.
5) Motivate yourself with a friend or a small group of friends who are also committed to a healthy lifestyle.
6) Keep a food journal for at least three to six months, until your new healthy ways are a habit.
7) Think about what you are about to eat five minutes before your meal so you make more conscious choices.
8) Place a sign on your refrigerator, which says, "If I'm not hungry, I don't eat."
9) Avoid eating after 7 p.m.
10) Clean all of the sugary products out of your kitchen.
11) Have at least five sugarless snacks available for travel, work and home.
12) Learn to cook and teach your kids how to cook.

General plan:
1. No sugary drinks, no diet drinks
2. 6 to 8 glasses of water daily
3. 30-50% less fructose
4. No more than 2-3 pieces of fruit daily
5. 50% vegetables, 25% of 100% complex carbs, 25% lean organic meat, nuts and seeds
6. Detox for two weeks
7. Exercise for 30 minutes five days a week, lift weights three days a week
8. Avoid dairy products
9. Avoid wheat if gluten sensitive

Rules
1) If it has a label, don't eat it (or at least learn to read the label).
2) Avoid food in a box or package
3) Don't add salt
4) Stay away from deadly white flour and sugar products
5) Know the fructose content of your food-see table back of the book
6) Avoid any food that has high fructose corn syrup in it
7) Avoid all sweeteners
8) No diet drinks
9) Throw out any food with preservatives, additives, coloring or dies or natural flavors like MSG.
10) Eat organic foods without hormones, pesticides and other chemicals.
11) Lean meat or fish should be organic-not from a pond or from concentrated animal feeding organizations.

12) Use only plant oils sparingly olive or coconut oil.
13) Increase intake of dark, green, leafy vegetables, including spinach, collard greens, turnip greens, mustard greens, vegetables that grow in the ground, cabbage, green beans, squash, cauliflower, onions, mushrooms.
14) Limited intake of saturated fat and primarily use mono saturated fats, olives, avocados, nuts and seeds. Eliminate animal products (meat and dairy).
15) Eat fruit low on the glycemic index, 2 to 3 pieces daily at most.
16) Limit fructose intake to around 35 grams daily.

Enjoy the following foods:
non-starchy veggies-low glycemic index foods
asparagus
bell peppers
broccoli
cauliflower
collard greens
cucumbers
green beans
kale
spinach
zucchini

Proteins:
beans
chicken
eggs
fish

lentils
nuts
seeds
turkey

Starchy foods:
beets
brown or black rice
carrots
buckwheat
corn
quinoa
sweet potatoes
turnips
winter squash

Low glycemic fruit:
apples
blackberries
blueberries
gogi berries
plums
kiwi
nectarines
peaches
raspberries
fruits with stones (seeds)

The Secrets

FOLLOWING ARE SEVERAL SECRETS TO a healthy diet and lifestyle that will help you along the way:

1) All carbohydrates are not alike. Starchy, complex carbohydrates quell hunger and turn up our internal furnace, burning calories as heat and energy. High sugar, high fat, simple carbohydrates increase hunger, food addictions and cravings.

2) The same starchy carbohydrates that prevent disease and premature death stop and even reverse disease.

3) The resistant starch in complex carbohydrates absorbs fat and cholesterol, while providing few calories and the feeling of fullness.

4) Refined carbohydrates reduce the "good" HDL cholesterol and increase insulin levels, triglycerides, blood pressure and fat stores-proven culprits in the development of inflammation, obesity, and diabetes and vascular disease.

5) Foods that promote weight loss are high in complex carbohydrates, which take more energy, calories, to break down. A faster metabolism and burn excess body fat.

6) Consumption of complex carbohydrates helps the brain produce higher levels of serotonin, which reduces your appetite and increases your feelings of well-being.

7) Reducing saturated fat without reducing refined carbo-hydrates works against the goal to lose weight and prevent or reverse chronic disease.

8) Saturated fats increase water clogging LDL cholesterol. The unsaturated fats and fish, flax seeds and plant-based oils reduce LDL cholesterol, inflammation and plaque within blood vessels.

9) Trans fat offer what the Mayo Clinic calls "a cholesterol double whammy" by raising "bad" LDL-cholesterol and lowering "good" HDL-cholesterol. The greater the percentage of trans fat in a food product, the higher risk for heart attacks and strokes.

10) Try to limit olive and other cooking oils while trying to lose weight, and then use them sparingly. Fish, ground flax seeds and walnuts offer the benefits of omega-3 fatty acids without all the fat of oil.

11) Animal protein raises cholesterol while plant protein lowers it. Meat also raises it.

12) To get the mental amount of protein you need each day, balance your vegetables with legumes and some nuts.

13) To lose weight faster, choose raw foods such as apples, carrots, bell peppers and other whole foods and vegetables eaten raw. Snacking on crunchy foods slows the rate of digestion and provides thousands of disease-fighting nutrients.

14) It takes 30 to 40 calories a day to maintain one pound of muscle. The more lean body mass you have, the faster your metabolism will be, and the greater number of calories you burn at rest. Do some weight training every week.

15) The same starchy carbohydrates that promote weight loss can prevent, stop and even reverse disease.
16) Eat a diet of foods containing vitamins, minerals and phytochemicals; it is the rainbow, symphony and mosaic of these that leads to good health.

Examples of Fructose Content in Fruits

FRUIT	Serving Size	Grams of Fructose
Limes	1 medium	0
Lemons	1 medium	0.6
Cranberries	1 cup	0.7
Passion fruit	1 medium	0.9
Prune	1 medium	1.2
Apricot	1 medium	1.3
Guava	2 medium	2.2
Dates	1 medium	2.6
Cantaloupe	1/8 of med. melon	2.8
Raspberries	1 cup	3.0
Clementine	1 medium	3.4
Kiwifruit	1 medium	3.4
Blackberries	1 cup	3.5
Star fruit	1 medium	3.6
Cherries sweet	10	3.8
Strawberries	1 cup	3.8
Cherries sour	1 cup	4.0
Grapefruit	1/2 medium	4.3
Boysenberries	1 cup	4.6
Nectarine	1 medium	5.4

Peach	1 medium	5.9
Orange	1 medium	6.1
Papaya	1/2 medium	6.3
Honeydew	1/8 of med. melon	6.7
Banana	1 medium	7.1
Blueberries	1 cup	7.4
Apple	1 medium	9.5
Watermelon	1/16 med. melon	11.3
Pear	1 medium	11.8
Raisins	1/4 cup	12.3
Grapes	1 cup	12.4
Mango	1/2 medium	16.2
Figs, dried	1 cup	23.0

Summary

WE NOW KNOW SUGAR IS the main cause of obesity, abdominal obesity, and non-alcoholic fatty liver disease, type II diabetes, vascular disease, hypertension, autoimmune disease, a leading cause of cancer, autoimmune disease and the other chronic illnesses.

Glucose and fructose in excess are the main problem. They are both toxic, the evil twins and fructose being the main culprit. Fructose is recognized differently in the body because of its configuration, its molecules are arranged slightly different, but there is still the same amount of atoms in both. There are 6 carbon atoms, 12 hydrogen atoms and 6 oxygen atoms, which is why they have the same chemical formula ($C_6H_{12}O_6$), but they are arranged in different shapes - fructose is pentagon-shaped and glucose is hexagon-shaped.

The scientific literature clearly reveals now that fructose is largely metabolized in the liver, soaking up your ATP, causes insulin and leptin resistance and results in a lot of chronic illness.

You can see the importance of knowing the sugar, glucose, and fructose content of your foods; that is critical.

Don't get fooled by the term "oh it's natural sugar" like what I heard a mother say at my grandson's tennis tournament yesterday. She was speaking about the little drinks in a plastic bag that the little kids just loved, I immediately responded by saying that must be the sugar in them, although I was not familiar with the drink. Sure enough, my three-year-old grandchild of mine had just drunk this little item and it had 11 grams of sugar. As usual someone had figured out the bliss point.

So it's glucose and fructose. If what you're drinking or eating is fructose, that doesn't mean it's low glucose. Both are evil and you need to know the content of both.

You can find out the fructose content of food and the back of the book of Dr. Richard Johnson called "Sugar Fix," a great read from which I quote liberally. Dr. Robert Lustig confirms most of the information in "Fat Chance."

You can learn about the sugar, glucose and fructose content of foods from the USDA website; they use nutrient analysis software created by research and food manufacturers.

I recommend you start with a 2 to 4 week period of detoxification from glucose and fructose. Meanwhile, educate yourself extensively about nutrition, especially the sugars. Just reading this book will give you a great start. Be sure to read the labels and know what they say. It'll get to be a habit

Exercise regularly if you can, even a half-hour walk daily is satisfactory. You can also dance in place and do some lightweights.

Also, learn about" sitting disease" also called NEAT, none exercise activity thermodynamics. You can watch my video on YouTube, using my last name that explains it in more detail. In essence you can burn a lot of calories by increasing your calorie burn in doing the routine activities in your life. For example if you can increase your calorie burn by 200 calories a day, through many different methods, you would have a 20-pound weight loss end of the year. It's about increasing your calorie burn in your "none exercise activities" which can result in a lot of weight loss over time and lead to good health.

SUMMARY

We are a nation under sugar and need to be educated and informed to reduce our international epidemic of obesity and its unfortunate complications. Remember sugar is as addictive and powerful as cocaine.

We need to reset our sugar thermostat, we need to detox.

Don't eat a sugary breakfast, pack it with good protein. Don't use sugar for quick fix. Learn about good snacks and have them available for your children also. No sugar drinks, no diet drinks, drink water with lemon.

Eat foods with flavoring, full of phytochemicals.

Enjoy and love your family. Learn about proper sleep and exercise as this can prevent a lot of disease. Don't treat your stress with America's favorite stress reliever, sugar.

Be sure you know the 50 or so names for other types of sugar, like corn syrup, corn starch, lactose, maltose, etc.

Wake up your taste buds, and lower your blood sugar with nutrient-dense foods.

By using spices you can crush a lot of cravings.

Lastly, you must pay attention every day to sugar consumption, glucose and fructose. Make a good breakfast. Stay ahead of "sugar creep" and be vigilant. Plan your treats to be mindful of what you're eating daily. Plan your day so you don't backslide.

Lastly develop habits they give you as much joy as "the sugar fix."

Good luck!

MORE RESOURCES FROM RUDY KACHMANN M.D.

Also visit Dr. Kachmann's YouTube channel www.youtube.com/drrudykachmann

Books:
Fructose – The Evil Twin
The Golden Opportunity
Narcotics: The Highway To Hell
Pain: We Need a New Definition
The Fraud of Chronic Pain
Healing Cancer with The Power Of Your Mind
Live to Be 100 with a Sound Mind and Body
The Call of Life
The Fraud of Alzheimer's Disease (also available on DVD)
Nocebo: Placebo's Evil Twin (also available on DVD and CD)
The Secret of the Non Diet for Adults (also available on DVD and CD)
The Secret of the Non Diet for Children (also available on DVD and CD)
Kid Scripts: Just What the Doctor Ordered
The Psychology of Eating (also available on DVD and CD)
Reversing Type 2 Diabetes in 60 Days (also available on DVD and CD)
Welcome to Your Mind Body (also available on DVD and CD)
Secrets of Motivating Yourself to Wellness (also available on DVD and CD)
For more titles, visit www.amazon.com.

DVDs:

The Mind and Stress (also available on CD)
Living Healthier and Longer (also available on CD)
Chinese Medicine (also available on CD)
Acute and Chronic Pain (also available on CD)
Smoking Cessation (also available on CD)
True Vitality (DVD only)
Secrets of the Mind and Cancer (DVD only)

For more titles, visit www.amazon.com.

www.ingramcontent.com/pod-product-compliance
Lightning Source LLC
Chambersburg PA
CBHW070303290526
45791CB00003B/1066